Good Sleep Is Essential

James Williams

DISCLAIMER

This information is provided and sold with the knowledge that the publisher and author do not offer any legal or other professional advice. In the case of a need for any such expertise consult with the appropriate professional. This book does not contain all information available on the subject. This book has not been created to be specific to any individual's or organizations' situation or needs. Every effort has been made to make this book as accurate as possible. However, there may be typographical and or content errors. Therefore, this book should serve only as a general guide and not as the ultimate source of subject information. This book contains information that might be dated and is intended only to educate and entertain. The author and publisher shall have no liability or responsibility to any person or entity regarding any loss or damage incurred, or alleged to have incurred, directly or indirectly, by the information contained in this book.

Thank you for downloading this book. Please review on Amazon for us so that I can make future versions even better. A portion of the proceeds from this book goes to American Cancer Society®. Thank you for you support. God bless.

Just for Downloading this book and showing your support, I wanna give you 2 of our other books, absolutely **FREE**. Just go to the link and subscribe and get **2 Free Books** for your support. Don't forget to give us **5 star Rating** so we can make better versions to help more people. Thank you guys for your support.

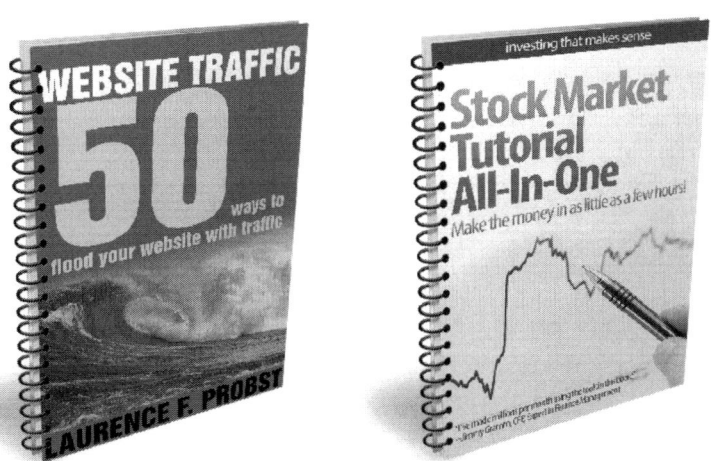

Click Here to Download-Free **Website Traffic & How To Invest in The Stock Market**

Table of Contents

Foreword 7

1. Cut Down Media Time Before Hitting The Hay 9

2. Physical Exercise For Better Sleep 13

3. Use Foods To Sleep Better 17

4. Jump On The Power Nap 23

5. Better Your Sleep With Visualization 29

6. Progressive Muscle Relaxation For Better Sleep 33

7. Utilize Relaxation Response 37

8. Use Aromatherapy 41

9. Does Sleep Really Affect Productivity 45

Wrapping Up 51

Foreword

Nothing shoots down your ability to get affairs done faster than a foul night's sleep. Surveys show that sleep deprivation costs Americans substantial work productiveness; yawning employees can't remain alert, make beneficial decisions, center on tasks or even negotiate a friendly mood at the office or with clients. There are lots of ways to crush insomnia, step-up the quality of your slumber, and master the power nap. This book will provide favorite sleep strategies, ideas and facts.

Chapter 1:

Cut Down Media Time Before Hitting The Hay

Synopsis

Utilizing a light emitting device Before hitting the hay like a fluttering TV set or computer monitor arouses the brain in a different way than the way the body was meant to move toward sleep (bit by bit like sundown) That's how come it is so simple to cast-off sleepless hours flicking from channel to channel. The exposure to light arouses the brain and brings on a false alertness and stimulus.

Turn It Off

Lay off checking your e-mail or watching television just before hitting the hay and you'll sleep more effectively. A recent field of study establishes that individuals who run through electronic media (read: stare at a backlit screen) just prior to bedtime report lower-quality slumber even when they acquire as much sleep as non-pre-bedtime media-heads.

This isn"t just bunk as a field of study at Osaka University in Japan demonstrated that individuals who surf the net or keep an eye on television prior to bedtime report that they're not getting adequate slumber—all the same, they're capturing as many Z's as individuals who don't view television or surf prior to going to bed.

The longer media utilization before slumber can touch off (self-perceived) deficient sleep," lead research worker Dr. Nakamori Suganuma, of Osaka University, Japan, said. So cyberspace and television utilization alters "sleep demand and sleep quality." It's time to switch off that computer well in front of bedtime, people.

I chanced upon this not too long ago. If I keep an eye on television or work at the computer inside about 2 hours of bedtime, I can't get to sleep. It's worse than taking in caffeine, for me. So now I have a self enforced "bedtime" for the computer and the television set, and I commonly spend the last hour approximately before hitting the hay reading a book. It's made all the difference in the world for me.

Try out the experiment yourself. If you're reading this e-book you in all likelihood spend a mess of time on the computer like I do. Quit using the computer a couple of hours prior to hitting the hay and as bed time draws near bring down the level of lighting in your home using more mood lighting than task lighting. Reading prior to bed won't damage sleep, it occupies a different part of the brain than studying off a brightly lit monitor does. You'll discover you're much sleepier and it's more comfortable to doze off.

I've recently embarked on reading for an hour prior to sack time. The time I hit the sack hasn"t switched, but I feel so a great deal better in the morning as a result.

As well, once a while go electronic-free, switch off all the electric-powered stuff in your home (perhaps shut out the light and fans/ heaters, etc) have a calm meals, talk to your loved ones then hit the hay. Uh-huh! EMR minimal, and maximized sleep or rest.

Chapter 2:

Physical Exercise For Better Sleep

Synopsis

You already recognize that working out provides bunches of healthiness benefits—a beneficial night's sleep being among them. But make certain you do the right kind of exercise at the right time of day.

Get Moving

The National Sleep Foundation says that physical exercise in the afternoon can assist in deepened shut-eye and abbreviate the time it takes for you to fall into sleepy-sleepy land. However, they caution, vigorous work outs leading up to bedtime may in reality have the inverse effects.

Quality Sleep

A study from a few years back found that a morning time fitness regimen was key to a better slumber. Research workers at the Fred Hutchinson Cancer Research Center resolved that postmenopausal adult females who worked out half-hour every morning had less trouble dozing off than those who were active to a lesser extent. The adult females who worked out in the evening hours saw small or no betterment in their sleep patterns. Oh sure, exercise heightens that other bedtime action, too: sex. (But that's a whole topic.)

Exercise has so many tension management and wellness benefits, and for many of us, night is when it best fits our schedules. Light exercise like yoga or taking a walk at night can likewise assist sleep as it releases stress without over stimulating the body. (It"s arguable whether or not "light" exercise right before bed disrupts sleep; according to sports medicine expert Elizabeth Quinn, it could in reality better sleep).

Yoga, which gains its name from the word, "yoke"—to draw together— does just that, drawing together the mind, body and spirit. But whether you practice yoga for spiritual transformation or for tension management and physical welfare or sleep, the advantages are many. The use of yoga involves stretching out the body and shaping different poses, while maintaining breathing as slow and controlled. The body gets relaxed and energized at the same time. There are assorted styles of yoga, some propelling through the poses more quickly, almost like an aerobic exercise, and other styles unwinding deeply into each pose. A few have a more spiritual tilt, while others are utilized purely as a sort of exercise.

Almost everybody can see physical benefits from yoga, and its use can likewise give psychological benefits, like stress reduction and a sense of welfare, and spiritual benefits, like a feeling of connection with God or Spirit, or a feeling of transcendency. Particular poses can be done almost anyplace and a yoga program can go for hours or minutes, depending upon one"s schedule.

Another thing to look into is Qigong. There are many ways Qigong can assist you to sleep soundly and more deeply. It"s an first-class "stress reducer". And as it is so simple to learn and easy to practice, it's rather easy to reserve a couple of minutes before bed time to execute this relaxing routine.

Quality Sleep

Tension reduction is an instant result of rehearsing Qigong and additionally there are other advantages. Qigong might be practiced standing, sitting, lying down or walking, consequently, for those of you that have trouble slumbering due to habitual pain, even back pain, Qigong can help here also. Maybe stress, anxiety or depression delivers reasons for your sleeplessness. If so, Qigong can help. It will equalize the body"s energy scheme and gently help the self-healing of nearly any complaint. The simple motions of qigong are often more comfortable to perform than the postures and stances in yoga. There are a lot of books and resources available to get you going with your qigong routine.

Chapter 3:

Use Foods To Sleep Better

Synopsis

A few foods are more tributary to an improved night's sleep than others. You already have heard about warm milk, chamomile tea and turkey, but there are others, like bananas, potatoes, oatmeal and brown bread. You find yourself driving back afternoon sagging eyelids? Here are a few pointers on eating foods to better sleep.

Yes… I'm Telling You To Eat Sleep inducing foods:

Foods high in tryptophan are beneficial sleep aids. Prior to hitting the sack, try one or more of the following foods to assist you in sleep. The basic denominator in these foods is that they contain tryptophan which has been demonstrated to assist sleep:

- Sesame seeds
- Spirolina
- Spinach
- Bananas
- Figs
- Dates
- Soy
- Turkey
- Silken Tofu

Turkey

Get a mental picture of granddad last Thanksgiving Day: at rest on the couch, head back, belt open -and it was only six p.m. It's not his 80 years it's the turkey. Turkey holds tryptophan, an aminoalkanoic acid that turns to the sleep - advancing neurotransmitter serotonin. To feel the turkey sleep enhancer, try eating a turkey sandwich 60 minutes before bedtime.

Warm milk

Equivalent to turkey, milk bears tryptophan, and the calcium and magnesium in milk assist and enhance the transition of tryptophan to serotonin. As for whether there's any reality to the old story about warm milk's slumber - causing powers, there is no study out yet.

I've heard for a long time that warming the milk makes the tryptophan more bioavailable to the body. However no one has ever executed a clinical study on warm milk vs. cold milk. If the idea of warm milk makes you feel all warm and fuzzy inside, apply it. If it makes you want to gag, gulp it cold. Either direction, try out a glass an hour prior to bedtime.

Prevent these foods prior to bedtime as they've been demonstrated to interrupt sleep patterns:

- Intoxicants
- Sugar
- Sauerkraut
- Cocoa
- Caffeine

Teas & herbaceous plants

A different option to prescription slumber aids are teas made from these herbaceous plants which have shown to be good as a natural slumber aid

- Nepeta cataria
- Hops
- Valerian root (which is in liquid or capsule forms)
- Passionflower vine (brew with chamomile)
- Skullcap
- Chamaemelum nobilis

Good vitamin supplementations

In addition to sound foods, there are a measure of nutritional supplements that may also help remedy sleeplessness. Calcium has long been acclaimed as a natural slumber aid. Think of the advice to drink a warm cup of milk to get better sleep. You are able to get better results by taking 1000 mg of Calcium lactate, or 1500-2000 mg calcium chelate. If having calcium chelate, it"s suggested to take it in split up doses.

Try 1000 mg of Magnesium instead of prescription slumber aids. These supplementations are best taken after meals and at bedtime

Likewise helpful to get more beneficial slumber is B complex plus extra pantothen; Inositol, and B6. Always observe the label recommendations.

Try out L-theanine aminoalkanoic acid.

This is a fantastic slumber aid! While L-theanine doesn't bring on sleep it does calm the "engaged mind" and does bring on alpha rhythm activity in the brain. (It's among the ingredients listed in Melissa, an all natural slumber aid.) This free form aminoalkanoic acid, gained from green tea, quiets and relaxes without side effects.

Additional conditions to get more beneficial slumber.

- A different cause of insomnia may include copper and iron inadequacies in adult females. A hair analysis ought to be done to ascertain if such inadequacies are present.

- Fresh air, melatonin, decompressing with a book, calming music, and a regular schedule are likewise effectual natural slumber aids.

- Yoga and other loosening techniques help clear the mind and abbreviate stress, preparing the body for sleep.

- Make sure to visit your physician to eliminate any rudimentary physical condition that might preclude you from sleeping.

Chapter 4:

Jump On The Power Nap

Synopsis

Slowly but certainly, the advantages of the classic, 20-minute power nap are acquiring more acknowledgement, with big companies setting up sleep pods at the office and more software applications like Pzizz assisting to set the right power nap aural scene. Here's how to get the perfect nap.

10 Minutes Of Bliss

Candidly, although it's often mocked, the power nap is among the best tools for busy individuals who have to rely on clearness of thought in order to be the most effectual at what they do. T Basically if virtually all of your work involves thinking and wiggling your fingers on a keyboard, blackboard, or waving a writing utensil over a notepad then this most probably applies to you.

What are the rewards of power naps?

A power nap can cause the difference between a beneficial idea and a eminent idea. It can enhance relationships, both personal and professional; by letting you better center on a individual or group of individuals, their message, and enhances your ability to correctly act upon the newly received info.

What precisely is a power nap?

A power nap is a curt nap, commonly between 10 and 30 minutes long, assumed in the midst of the day in order to invigorate you for the next part of the day. Power naps are not like steady sleep, so you won"t be dazed after taking one. While you may have "dreams", power naps are more related to meditation, where thoughts are permitted to move from the subconscious to the conscious mind and back again without you centering on them. Power naps can be assumed just about anywhere where you are able to fully and honestly relax. The key is that it must be someplace mentally comfy.

Physical comfort is likewise crucial, but without the mental solace, the power nap looses its effect. This is why someplace private is pivotal to the successful power nap.

Ok, so how do you power nap?

To begin, find a location where you are able to nap uninterruptedly for at least ten minutes, or for the duration of your power nap. Switch off the lights and, if you wish, put on something restful (or boring) to listen to. You might as well wish to put some sort of an alarm on. Remember to give yourself at least a minute to emerge from the nap process.

Note: One crucial thing to remember is that the longer you sleep, the deeper you"ll go, and the more potential you"ll be groggy when you awaken.

Audio and Lighting

Audio: If you"ve had a particularly troubled day, or if you suffer from tinnitus, it might be helpful to have some kind of noise in the background which you are able to both lock on to and push aside at the same time. That"s since if you had such a day, then relaxing your mind might take too long, or be almost impossible, unless there's some sound there to focus on. This may be executed with both music and spoken text.

Lighting: This is in reality a bit of a touchy matter. Most individuals urge finding a dark, comfortable place. All the same, that"s more of a personal matter. If you"re power napping out of doors by a lake then you plainly can"t turn the sun off. Also, you might be in an office where you're unable to control the lighting. Or you might not mind the light at all, or even prefer it over dark. Or you may merely be among those folks who don"t care either way. Anyway, make certain you know what lighting situation is better for you and find a way to get into that prior to beginning your nap.

When you"ve discovered a place, make your self comfy by lying down and loosening your body. It's crucial that you lay facing up, even if you"re a side- or stomach-sleeper, as this pose will keep your back in suitable alignment and will make it easier for your body to speedily unwind. Ensure that your shoulders and arms are totally relaxed.

From this spot it"s all in your head, literally. The enticement here will be to start thinking of something, anything, actively. Don"t! If an idea comes to your mind, that"s fine, let it be there, but don"t center on it; don"t sustain it. Merely let it come and go.

Center on your breathing. Center on how your nostrils feel when air draws in and out, or how the air feels when it hits the back of your throat. If you're playing something, center on the sound of the instruments or voice, but don"t center on the tune, or what"s being said. Keep doing that as long as you require. This way, no idea can take root, and your mind will start to unload info faster. It might seem that your mind is now full and that you"re considering too much, but remember that you"re not thinking about anything, ideas are just passing. Your mind is now discharging information, and this is precisely what you want it to do.

Quickly you should almost feel like you"re beginning to dream. You might, in fact, do so. That"s o.k.. It means you"re at ease and your mind is refreshing itself.

Quality Sleep

If you've an alarm, when it goes off, merely open your eyes and lay there. Your alarm shouldn't be too intrusive. You don"t want to frighten yourself out of your nap. Most mobile phones have alarm features which will serve this purpose. Center on your breathing and open your eyes. Feel your body and begin to stretch along. sit up easy and take it all in. Your mind should be clear now.

Chapter 5:

Better Your Sleep With Visualization

Synopsis

There's nothing sorrier than lying awake throughout the nighttime, watching the clock tick away instants knowing you'll be the living dead the next day. When insomnia's booting you in your sleepy headed butt, use a self-directed meditative visualization strategy to quiet the whizz of a racing mind.

See Relaxation

Here"s a quieting visual image exercise to try out:

Sit down or lie down in a comfy position. Take in a deep breath. Picture that the earth below you has became blue, as bluish as the sky higher up. The ground below you is blue down as far as you are able to look.

Straight off see energy grooves spreading out on the underside of your feet. As you breathe in, visualize the blue colouring of the earth filling up your feet. Your breath is pulling in the color blue in from the ground like blue-colored Kool-Aid through a drinking straw. As your feet start to fill with the color blue, you breathe out blue air from your lungs by your mouth and nose. And as you breathe out this blue air, you sense that it is carrying away stress and tiredness from your body. Stress and weariness simply go away into the air.

As you go forward to breathe in this delightful blue color, it oozes into every muscle, every cell of your ankle joint, your calf muscle, your knee joint, your thigh muscle, up to your hip joint, your abdomen, and your chest.

At the same time blue breath is getting breathed out from your lungs, carrying off all the tenseness, all the anxiousness, all the stress, and all the weariness from your body.

The cool blue color is like a shot filling your arm muscles, your shoulder joints, your neck, your face, and your head.

Every bone in your body is full of loosening, quieting bluish color. All the stress and weariness has left your body. Zero stays on but cool, quiet, unwinding, luxurious blue. Relish in the glorious blue color for as long as you care to. Then allow it to vaporize from every pore of your body, allowing you to feel relaxed, freshened up, and totally at rest.

Visualization is one strategy that utilizes the might of your mind to help naturally mend your body. Exercises like this one work best when you're in an unstrained state. Attempt them during meditation, self-suggestion, or yoga.

Chapter 6:

Progressive Muscle Relaxation For Better Sleep

Synopsis

Progressive Muscle Relaxation (PMR) is a bang-up strategy for reducing total body tension and getting better sleep. As you rehearse tensing and relaxing all the muscle groups in your body, you are able to move to a abbreviated procedure, Deep Muscle Relaxation where you quickly unwind your whole body. As you come down the tension you carry in your body, your whole being will feel less tension and you'll enjoy increased physical and emotional health as well as better slumber. Here's how to get going.

Relax All Of It

The physical component calls for the tensing and relaxing of muscle groups over the arms, legs, face, stomach and chest. With the eyes shut and in a successive pattern, a tension in a given muscle group is purposefully caused for approximately ten seconds and then discharged for twenty seconds before going along with the next muscle group.

The mental component centers on the difference between the feelings of the tension and relaxation. As the eyes are shut, one is impelled to center on the sensation of tension and relaxation. In persons with anxiousness, the mind often thinks "I don't know if this will work" or "Am I experiencing it yet." If such is the case, the person is told to simply center on the feelings of the tensed up muscle. Because of the feelings of warmth and weightiness are felt in the relaxed muscle after it's tensed up, a mental relaxation is experienced as a result.

1. Once you have found a quiet place and a few free minutes to rehearse progressive muscle relaxation, sit down or lie down and make yourself easy.

2. Start out by tensing up all the muscles in your face. Constitute a tight grimace, shut your eyes as tightly as conceivable, clinch your teeth, even move your ears up if you are able to. Carry on this part for the count of 8 as you breathe in.

3. Now breathe out and loosen up entirely. Let your face go totally loose, as if you were sleeping. Feel the tautness ooze from your facial muscles, and delight in the feeling.

4. Following, wholly tense up your neck and shoulders, once again breathing in and counting to 8. Then breathe out and loosen up.

5. Carry on down your body, duplicating the routine with the following muscle groups:

   - Chest
   - Stomach
   - Total right arm
   - Right forearm and hand (establishing a fist)
   - Right hand
   - Total left arm
   - Left forearm and hand (once again, establishing a fist)

- Left hand
- Buttocks
- Total right leg
- Lower right leg and foot
- Right foot
- Total left leg
- Lower left leg and foot
- Left foot

6. For the abbreviated variation, which lets in just 4 chief muscle groups:

- Face
- Neck, shoulders and arms
- Stomach and chest
- Buttocks, legs and feet

Rapidly centering on each group one after the other, with rehearsal you are able to relax your body like "liquified relaxation" poured out on your head and it flowed down and totally covered you. You are able to use progressive muscle relaxation to rapidly de-stress any time as well as to ready your body for a good nights sleep.

Chapter 7:

Utilize Relaxation Response

Synopsis

The relaxation response is a state that's opposite to the tension response. Practitioners of Transcendental Meditation claim they can lower their blood pressure with this technique.

Another Relaxation Method

Upon being studied it was found that practicers of this technique could slow their breathing by twenty-five percent, diminish their oxygen consumption by seventeen percent, lower their blood pressure, and slow down their pulse rate.

In order to make the technique more approachable and scientific, researchers removed the Eastern religious factor and condensed the basic strategy of Transcendental

Meditation, which is said to be a component of every major religious tradition or meditative pattern— the repeating of a word, sound, prayer, or phrasal idiom to the exclusion of other thinking.

Nowadays, this technique helps individuals manage the negative effects of stress and reduce stress-related symptoms as well as improve their sleep.

How to accomplish the strategy:

1. Discover a calm and quiet place and sit down in a comfy position. Attempt to loosen up all your muscles.

2. Shut your eyes.

3. Select a word, phrase, or prayer to center on that has particular meaning to you, is securely rooted in your belief system, or makes you feel at peace a few examples are "one", "serenity", "I am with you Lord", "I am one with the universe", or even a word like "thankful".

4. Take a breath slowly and naturally. Breathe in through your nose and hesitate for a couple of seconds. Breathe out

through your mouth, once again hesitating for a couple of seconds. Wordlessly say your focus word, phrase, or prayer as you breathe out.

5. Do not concern yourself about how well you are doing and do not feel badly if thoughts or feelings trespass in your mind. Merely say to yourself "Oh well" and go back to your repeating.

6. When the time comes to the end, remain aware of your breathing but sit down quietly. Getting aware of where you are, slowly open up your eyes and rise bit by bit.

This strategy is generally practiced for ten to twenty minutes per day, or at the least 3 to 4 times a week.

If you have to keep track of the time, try utilizing an alarm or timer set on the smallest volume, so you don't have to keep viewing your watch or clock.

Stress can cause severe wellness problems and, in extreme cases, can induce death. While stress management techniques have been shown to have a positive effect on reducing stress and bettering sleep, they're for guidance only, and readers should take the advice of fittingly qualified health care providers if they have any concerns over stress-related illnesses or if stress is causing significant or persistent unhappiness and loss of sleep.

Chapter 8:

Use Aromatherapy

Synopsis

Aromatherapy is generally used to facilitate stress relief, but it's as well useful in addressing sleep disorders. Aromatherapy is the therapeutic utilization of essential oils to comfort and mend, and it is among the fastest growing complementary therapies in the Western world.

Smell Your Way To Good Sleep

In aromatherapy, the essential oils are utilized topically instead of being taken internally. The essential oils are said to perk up an area of the brain, known as the limbic system that commands mood and emotion. Firm scientific backing for aromatherapy is deficient, but there's info, without doubt, that many individuals find it a soothing complement to other self-help measures to ease stress, promote relaxation behavior, and aid in sleep as part of their bedtime readyings. So you might prefer to give it a try.

To assist in restoring restful slumber, you are able to try utilizing essential oils one by one or in combination. The essential oils are typically available at health food stores, while these days many pharmacies as well carry a variety of the oils. The most normally advocated oil for promoting sleep is lavender, but there are a lot of others that may have a soothing effect.

Try out adding a couple of drops of essential oil to warm water for a unwinding bath or footbath, or spritz the oil onto a hankie or small pillow. You are able to as well utilize a few drops to a heat diffuser near your bed to disperse the scent through the room or use a particularly made ring that can be placed on the electric-light bulb of a bedside lamp; the heat of the bulb circulates the scent.

You may as well prefer to try blending the relaxing benefits of aromatherapy and massage by making your own scented massage oil. Dilute one to 3 drops of essential oil per teaspoonful of an unscented carrier oil, like almond or grapeseed oil. (Do not utilize undiluted essential oil by placing directly on to your skin.) Since some individuals are more sensitive to the oils than other people, begin with the littlest amount, and experiment till you determine the combination that works best for you.

Research is beginning to confirm lavender's tranquilizing qualities. It's been discovered to lengthen total sleep time, step-up deep sleep, and make individuals feel reinvigorated. It seems to work better for adult females, maybe because women tend to have a more intense olfactory modality.

The beneficial thing about lavender is that it starts to work quickly. Once again try placing a lavender sachet under your pillow or place one to two drops of lavender essential oil in a hankie. Or add several drops of lavender oil to a bath -- the drop in body temperature after a warm bath as well assists with better sleep.

You can as well make a sweet smelling sleep pillow.

Having a pleasant scent filling up your nostrils when you get into bed might help you drop off to dreamland. A perfumed pillow is one way to produce this effect. To create a scented pillow, you are able to, naturally, spray a little of essential oil onto your regular pillow. But you are able to as well create an herb-filled sleep pillow by mixing aromatic herbs and sewing them into a small piece of soft fabric. You'll want the pillow to be modest and flat, so you are able to slip it into your regular pillow slip, on top of your regular pillow. Here's a sweet but powerful mixture for an herbal pillow:

- 4 parts dried out lavender leaves
- 2 parts dried out hops
- 2 parts dried out rose petals
- 1 part dried out chamomile
- 1 part dried out lemon balm

The herbs finally lose their scent and ought to be replaced after about nine to twelve months.

Chapter 9:

Does Sleep Really Affect Productivity

Synopsis

Do you find yourself making more and bigger mistakes?

It Makes A Difference

You might never have blundered so dramatically, but the odds are you're not getting the 7 to 8 hours of nightly shuteye experts agree you require. While a few high-achieving entrepreneurs boast of taking minimal z's, research demonstrates that our sleep needs are astonishingly consistent. If you fail to get at least 7 nightly hours, you're likely operating at a cognitive disadvantage.

And your health and your business might be paying the price. Business owners seem to share a hefty ambivalence toward sleep, both craving and ostracizing it. That's particularly true in this bad economy - a recent poll found that small-business owners are working longer, thanks to the decline - and during a startup stage.

So what? You enquire. Aren't you more productive when you work eighteen hour days? Can't you just shore up your droopy eyelids by downing yet another cup of coffee?

Unfortunately, no. New scientific research demonstrates that going without enough sleep for more than an occasional day or two can play havoc on your wellness, memory, concentration, temper, and ability to arrive at decisions - even if you believe you're doing all right.

If you require a good reason to begin sacking out earlier or sleeping later, here it is. It turns out that far from being a time waster, sleep makes you fitter, smarter, and a more beneficial leader - and might even yield great thoughts for growing your business.

The evidence that sleep matters is incontrovertible and perpetually growing. Let's begin with a freshly discovered link between sleep loss and serious sicknesses like diabetes and cancer. A 2008 scientific research at the University of Chicago's school of medicine kept young, healthy volunteers alert for all but 4 hours a night for 6 nights running. The resultant: The levels of subjects' hormones shifted - particularly a hormone called leptin that bears on appetite. They got ravenously hungry, gulping down pizza and ice cream long after they'd have felt full generally, and their blood glucose shot up to pre-diabetic levels - an menacing result after less than one week of poor sleep.

Other analyses repeat those results so regularly that researchers now trust that not getting enough sleep is a lead cause of obesity and diabetes, both of which are on the rise across the country. At the same time, the WHO has accumulated data from around the Earth showing that sleep loss depresses the immune system, to the point where WHO is thinking about labeling chronic sleep loss a carcinogen, comparable to tobacco and asbestos.

If you've ever been so tired out that you had to reread the same paragraph several times to grip its meaning and soon blanked out what you read, you already know what sleep investigators have lately demonstrated about the effects of too little sack time on productivity.

One experiment at a school of medicine kept subjects up until four A.M., woke them at eight A.M., and then fed them a series of tests designed to measure memory, vigilance, and the ability to react quickly to fresh data. The researchers were startled to find that subjects' mental acuity slumped markedly after just one night and kept falling with each successive night of 4 hours' sleep. Even more distressing: The study's volunteers were incognizant of their deterioration. One woman, so tired that she could barely say her name, was all the same sure she was able to drive home.

Regardless how much you believe you're achieving when you pull an all-nighter, it's likely to a lesser degree than what you could accomplish if you got some sleep then returned to work. A study gave volunteers a list of words to memorize and then were kept alert for twenty-four hours, their power to recall the words fell by forty%. Memory betters during sleep, so that if you get a full 7 or 8 hours sleep tonight, your recall of all that happened today will be twenty% to thirty%

sharper than it is directly after the day's events happen. No one is for certain yet why this is so.

For entrepreneurs, the finest reason to get enough shuteye might be to avoid making dense, costly decisions. A sleep researcher recently gave 3 groups of subjects the same pieces of data. Those who walked off and spent at least 7 of the next 12 hours sleeping were able to brand broader and more lucid connections than those who didn't get much (or any) sleep or those who attempted to analyze the data right away.

A lot of successful CEOs discuss having good instincts. I'd argue that all they're doing is permitting themselves at least twelve hours to marinate the data they absorb - and if those twelve hours include some sleep, they get even finer results.

Wrapping Up

The more province you have, to a greater extent the lack of sleep hurts you. Entrepreneurs require more sleep than most individuals, not less, yet seldom acquire enough, particularly in these turbulent economical times. There's a mentality that values burning down the midnight oil. However once you recognize how it affects you, purposely depriving yourself of sleep is actually sort of dumb. So is not doing everything you can to get better sleep.

Hopefully this book has given you the tools to have a different look at acquiring a better nights sleep.

Made in the USA
San Bernardino, CA
24 April 2015